T0234273

Burning Mouth Disease

Isaäc van der Waal

Burning Mouth Disease

A Guide for Patients

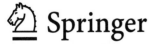 Springer

Isaäc van der Waal
Former head of the Department of
Oral Maxillofacial Surgery/Pathology
Amsterdam University Medical Center/
Academic Center for Dentistry (ACTA)
Amsterdam, The Netherlands

ISBN 978-3-030-94228-1   ISBN 978-3-030-94226-7   (eBook)
https://doi.org/10.1007/978-3-030-94226-7

This Springer imprint is published by the registered company Springer Nature
Switzerland AG
The registered company address is: Gewerbestrasse 11, 6330 Cham, Switzerland

Preface

Burning mouth disease (BMD), also referred to as burning mouth syndrome, is an enigmatic disease for both the patient and clinician. When the disease is not recognized as such, the patient may become exposed to a wide variety of redundant treatments, including dental and surgical procedures.

This guide is primarily written for patients suffering from BMD and BMD-like symptoms. The goals are to inform patients about the various aspects of their disease and to provide them with the tools to communicate with healthcare providers. It is the author's experience that proper patient information and empathy will often change an apparently unbearable disease into a more or less acceptable one to live with, thereby avoiding redundant dental or medical treatments, drug prescriptions, and referrals.

For dental and medical healthcare providers a more detailed monograph is available (Van der Waal I. Burning mouth disease; a guide to diagnosis and management. Springer, 2021. ISBN 978-3-030-71,639-4; eBook ISBN 978-3-030-71640-0).

The present text is largely based on the literature from the past decades and, above all, on personal experience with a vast number of BMD patients who have been referred to the Department of Oral and Maxillofacial Surgery/Oral Medicine/Oral Pathology of the VU Vrije Universiteit medical centre/ACTA, Amsterdam, the Netherlands. Where appropriate, terminologies when used for the first time are explained in a glossary.

Finally, I would like to express my gratitude to all employees of Springer Nature for their pleasant and efficient collaboration during the realization of this guide.

Amsterdam, The Netherlands   Isaäc van der Waal

Contents

About the Author

Isaäc van der Waal (1943), born in the Netherlands, is an emeritus professor of Oral Pathology at the dental and medical school of the Vrije Universiteit in Amsterdam, the Netherlands, and has been the head of the Department of Oral and Maxillofacial Surgery/Pathology. He has been trained in oral surgery, oral medicine, and oral pathology and is the author or co-author of more than 400 papers in peer-reviewed scientific journals. In addition, he wrote several books in the field of oral diseases. Isaäc van der Waal has over 45 years of experience in the management of patients suffering from burning mouth disease.

Introduction

1

1.1 Introduction

Burning mouth disease (BMD) is a rare but serious, chronic disease. It is not a disease of modern times and has been reported already in an historical review of the period 1800–1950 [1].

Patients suffering from BMD may consult not only their dentist or general practitioner but also various medical specialists, such as the otolaryngologist, the oral and maxillofacial surgeon, the dermatologist and the neurologist. Unfortunately, first-line healthcare providers often do not recognize the symptoms associated with BMD. As a result, patients may undergo unnecessary diagnostic tests and treatments, varying from drug prescriptions, extractions of teeth, to psychiatric treatment.

In this chapter, attention will be paid to the various terminologies, definitions, and classifications of BMD that are used in the literature. Furthermore, the epidemiology (see Glossary) of BMD will be discussed.

© The Author(s), under exclusive license to Springer Nature Switzerland AG 2022
I. van der Waal, *Burning Mouth Disease*,
https://doi.org/10.1007/978-3-030-94226-7_1

1.2   Terminology and Definition

1.2.1   Terminology

In the past, the term glossodynia has been used to describe a painful tongue, and the term glossopyrosis to describe a burning sensation in the tongue. When just discomfort is experienced, the term dysaesthesia (see Glossary) has been used. Likewise, for burning sensations elsewhere in the mouth, with or without involvement of the tongue, the terms stomatodynia (pain of the mouth), stomatopyrosis (burning of the mouth), and oral (see Glossary) dysaesthesia have been used. Other terminologies include 'burning mouth disorder' and, most commonly, 'burning mouth syndrome'. In the present text, preference is given to the term 'burning mouth disease' (BMD). The use of 'burning' in the terminology may be somewhat confusing for those patients in whom the complaints do not so much consist of burning but, instead, of itching, tingling, or bizarre sensations, such as a sandpaper sensation.

Denture-wearing patients may occasionally complain of a burning or itching sensation limited to the palate (roof of the mouth) underneath the upper denture. This condition is referred to as 'denture sore mouth' (DSM). In fact, DSM can be considered a subtype of BMD.

1.2.2   Definition

There is no internationally accepted definition of BMD. In the present text the following definition is used: *'an intraoral (see Glossary) burning or dysaesthetic sensation of normal looking oral mucosa (see Glossary), recurring daily, with or without associated symptoms such as dry mouth or taste disturbance'.*

The almost diagnostic symptoms of BMD are described in Chap. 2.

1.3 Classification

1.3.1 Classification Based on the Course of the Symptoms

Largely based on the course of the symptoms, some authors recognize three subtypes of BMD [2], being:

- Type (1) symptoms are not present on waking but arise and increase in severity as the day progresses, without preventing the patient from falling asleep.
- Type (2) symptoms are continuously present, all day from waking. According to these authors, type 2 BMD patients are the most difficult to treat successfully because a high proportion suffers from chronic anxiety.
- Type (3) patients have symptom-free days and may have symptoms at unusual sites such as the floor of the mouth, buccal (see Glossary) mucosa and throat. According to these authors, about 10% of BMD patients present this history, which in the past has been reported as 'atypical' burning mouth.

1.3.2 Classification Based on the Presence of Associated Oral Symptoms

In another suggested classification three types of BMD are recognized: (1) full-blown BMD (mucosal pain, disturbed taste, and dry mouth), (2) pain and disturbed taste, or pain and dry mouth, and (3) pain only [3].

1.3.3 Comment

The two classifications mentioned above may have some value in scientific studies, but are not really relevant for the management of BMD patients.

1.4 Epidemiology

At present, there are hardly any epidemiologic data available of the prevalence (see Glossary) of BMD among large populations in different parts of the world. In most studies, only the prevalence in selected populations has been reported, such as in patients from a general dental practice, or patients visiting a menopause clinic or a diabetic clinic (Table 1.1) [4–8]. Because of the diversity of the selected populations, the way the figures have been collected, e.g., by self-reported questionnaires or by face-to-face interviews, and the use of different definitions of BMD at the time of the reported studies, it is difficult to assess the prevalence in a population at large, comprising all ages and both genders. *An estimated overall prevalence of 0.01–0.02%, which equals 100–200 patients per one million population at large, seems to be a reasonable one. When calculated for women >60 years, an estimated prevalence of 0.05–0.10% results.*

Little is known about possible racial, geographic, and sociodemographic differences.

The mean age of BMD patients is approximately 60 years. BMD in men occurs at a lower age than in women. Occurrence in patients below the age of a somewhat arbitrarily cut off point of 30 years is exceptional. In most of the reported studies, there is a female–male predilection of at least 5:1.

Table 1.1 Reported prevalence of burning mouth disease in various populations in the world

Type of population	Number of participating subjects	Prevalence (%)
Adult population in the USA [4]	41,000	0.7
Adult population in Sweden [5]	1427	4
Menopause clinic in Finland [6]	3173	8.2
Diabetic clinic (Diabetes mellitus type 1 patients in the USA) [7]	371	3.2
Hospitalized elderly patients in China [8]	21,972	15.7

Because of the low prevalence of BMD, it should be no surprise that most people have never heard from this disease. This ignorance can result in a strong feeling of isolation by the patients from their friends and close relatives [9].

2.1 Introduction

In most patients suffering from burning mouth disease (BMD) the tongue is the main site of their complaints. In some patients the burning sensation is present all day, while in others the symptoms are not present on waking but arise and increase in severity as the day progresses.

Many patients with BMD also suffer from a dry mouth, an altered taste or a smell disorder. Other inconveniences may consist of gastrointestinal (see Glossary) and urogenital (see Glossary) complaints. Less common complaints consist of burning feet, restless legs and simultaneous burning of the mouth and the vulva.

2.2 Burning Sensation and Other Dysaesthesias of the Oral Mucosa

"In the morning she feels fine, has little or no problems, but in the late afternoon it gets worse and in the evening the burning sensation in her mouth becomes unbearable. Finally, she takes a tranquillizer and goes to bed. She complains of a bad taste which is why she does not eat very much. I hope I have made things clear and may contribute to a better understanding of my mother's problem." The quotation is from one of the many rather characteristic letters of patients, in this case the daughter of a patient, who took part in a written inquiry among patients who suffer from BMD. Burning mouth disease may embitter life for patients completely ("When this is staying on forever, life does not mean anything anymore to me"). Indeed, in several studies among BMD patients a distinct impaired general health and oral health related quality of life has been reported, either caused by the burning sensations or by the often associated complaint of xerostomia or loss of taste [10, 11].

Instead of burning, some BMD patients describe their symptoms as prickling, itching, tingling, or bizarre sensations, such as a sandpaper sensation.

2.2.1 Sites of Burning Sensations

In almost all BMD patients, the burning sensation occurs at both sides of the tongue or other parts of the mouth, the lips, or the throat. The anterior two-thirds of the tongue and the tip of the tongue are the most commonly affected sites. In Table 2.1 the sites of burning in 154 BMD patients are presented [12]. In that study, involvement of the lips was quite common, but only in association

Table 2.1 Sites of burning in 154 BMD patients [12]

Location	%
Tip of the tongue	71
Lateral borders of the tongue	46
Dorsum of the tongue	46
Lips	50
Buccal mucosa	21
Palate	46
Throat	19
Upper denture-bearing tissue	25
Lower denture-bearing tissue	19
Oral cavity and throat	7

with symptoms of the tongue. Furthermore, the floor of the mouth was not mentioned as a site of burning, while in another study on BMD patients, 13% of the patients complained of burning sensations in that specific site of the mouth [13].

Occasionally, the burning symptoms are limited to the hard palate (see Glossary); in case of the presence of an upper denture and in the absence of clinical mucosal changes, the term 'denture sore mouth' is used, as has been explained in the introductory chapter.

2.2.2 Course of Burning Sensations

In the majority of BMD patients, the symptoms are present every day over a period of several months or even years. In many patients the symptoms are not present on waking but arise and increase in severity as the day progresses, without preventing the patient from falling asleep at night. The intensity of pain and levels of disability at different times through the day have been assessed in a study from Spain [14]. The results showed that in almost all BMD patients pain and disability, indeed, increase as the day progresses. The authors concluded that circadian rhythm (the 'internal body clock') dysfunction may contribute to the course of BMD symptoms through the day.

In most BMD patients, the burning sensations decrease while eating meals, drinking cold beverages, using chewing gum, or while working or being distracted. Spicy or acidic food/liquids or alcoholic beverages, stress, and tiredness often intensify the burning sensation.

2.2.3 Duration of Burning Sensations

In various studies in the world one has looked at the duration of the disease. For instance, in a study of 5 years duration some 50% of the patients reported no change in their symptoms, 25% moderate improvement, 20% worsening, while only 5% reported a complete disappearance of their symptoms without any treatment [15]. Indeed, in many BMD patients the symptoms may last for many years and, in some, even lifelong.

2.2.4 Onset of Burning Sensations

The onset of the burning sensations may be gradually or suddenly, with or without a triggering event. In one study, 33% of the patients reported an adverse life event, such as a stillborn child, children injured in accidents or prolonged social problems, moving house or marital difficulty, as a possible triggering event [12]. In another study, the onset of BMD was related to a previous dental procedure in 33% of the patients and to a previous illness in 10%, while 57% of the patients could not relate the onset of their symptoms to any prior event (Table 2.2) [13]. Some patients may not disclose any adverse life events to their doctor or dentist, for instance for emotional reasons or lack of trust.

2.2.5 Patients' Delay

Little is known about the 'time lapse' between the first symptoms of BMD and the first consultation with the general practitioner or dentist. Probably, few BMD patients will avoid regular care, consulting alternative healthcare workers, instead. Patients tend not to disclose such information, being afraid to be humiliated. The same applies to the use of alternative drugs, e.g., herbal compounds.

Table 2.2 Onset of symptoms in BMD patients (in %)

Event	Van der Ploeg et al. [12]	Grushka [13]
Dental treatment	40	33
Medical treatment or illness	21	10
Adverse life events	33	–
Unknown	6	57

Table 2.3 Specialists consulted by BMD patients, apart from the dentist and the general practitioner [16]

Specialist	Number (n = 17)
Internist	8
Neurologist	6
Dermatologist	6
Otolaryngologist	5
Oral (maxillofacial) surgeon	4
Allergologist	4
Gynaecologist	4
Psychiatrist	3
Ophthalmologist	3
Total	43

2.2.6 Professional Diagnostic Delay

First-line healthcare providers often do not recognize the symptoms associated with BMD. As a result, the number of specialists consulted, apart from the dentist and the general practitioner, may be up to three or even more, often referred to as the 'healthcare journey' of a patient [16]. An example of a small group of patients is shown in Table 2.3. Such patients may have been subjected to several unsuccessful and sometimes irreversible treatments for their complaints. These treatments vary from drug prescriptions, extractions of teeth, to psychiatric treatment.

2.3 Dry Mouth

A dry mouth may be either based on a subjective feeling of dryness ('xerostomia') in the presence of a more or less normal salivary flow, or on an objectively measured decrease of salivary flow ('hyposalivation'). The relevance of measuring the salivary flow is of limited value and is not performed routinely in BMD patients. The terms xerostomia and hyposalivation are often used intermingled. In the present text just the term xerostomia is used. Xerostomia is among the most common reported BMD-associated symptoms, being noticed in about 50–60% of BMD patients [13].

The feeling of dryness of the mouth is not necessarily related to a decreased salivary flow. Therefore, doctors and dentists should refrain from saying to a patient complaining of a dry mouth: "How can you suffer from a dry mouth? There is plenty of saliva".

2.4   Taste Disturbance

Complaints of ageusia (loss of taste) or dysgeusia (altered taste) may range from absence of taste to a bitter, sweet, salty, or metallic taste. There are several causes of taste disturbance, including a number of drugs, but in most cases the cause is unknown. Taste disturbances can also occur in patients suffering from BMD.

2.5   Smell Disorder

Smell disorders may vary from either complete loss of smell (anosmia) or decreased smell (hyposmia). In a study from Canada, 13% of BMD patients suffered from altered smell perception, compared to 8% in an age- and gender-matched control group [13].

2.6   Association with Other Orofacial Pain Disorders

2.6.1   Odontalgia

Toothache in one or more teeth for which no cause can be detected is called 'odontalgia'. There have been rare cases reported of odontalgia in BMD patients.

2.6.2   Temporomandibular Joint Complaints

In a small series of BMD patients, almost 70% showed signs and symptoms of temporomandibular joint disorders (see Glossary) [17].

2.7 Complaints Elsewhere in the Body

2.7.1 Common Complaints

In a study from Canada, the number of chronic pain complaints were compared between a group of BMD patients and a control group [13]. The number of chronic pains other than BMD was significantly higher for the BMD group than for the control group.

In a study from Italy, 98% of the BMD patients reported unexplained extraoral (see Glossary) symptoms [18]. The unexplained extraoral symptoms in BMD patients may consist of pain in different bodily areas, ear-nose-throat symptoms, neurological symptoms, ophthalmological (from the eyes) symptoms, gastrointestinal complaints, skin/gland complaints, urogenital complaints and cardiopulmonary symptoms.

2.7.2 Rare Complaints

2.7.2.1 Burning Feet
There are a few BMD patients reported who also complained about burning feet.

2.7.2.2 Parkinson's Disease
Studies on a possible relationship between Parkinson's disease and BMD have shown contradictory results.

2.7.2.3 Restless' Legs
A few BMD patients have been reported who also suffered from restless legs' syndrome.

2.7.2.4 Urological Diseases
The results of one study were suggestive of a possible association between BMD and urological (see Glossary) diseases.

2.7.2.5 Vulvodynia; Peno/Scrotodynia

There are a few reports on BMD patients who suffered from simultaneous burning of the mouth and the vulva ('vulvodynia'). There is a single BMD patient reported, who also suffered from peno/scrotodynia.

Perhaps these symptoms are more common among BMD patients, but may not be disclosed by the patients. It has been mentioned in the literature that patients seldom report genital symptoms to the dentist and dentists do not generally ask about genital symptoms.

2.7.2.6 Other Diseases That May Be Associated with Burning Mouth Disease

Numerous common and uncommon diseases in BMD patients have been reported in the literature [19]. Apart from anxiety (60%) and depression (50%), to be discussed in the next chapter, low back pain and neck and shoulder pain were the most common reported comorbidities (see Glossary), while life stressors were reported by more than 60% of the patients.

Suggested Causes of Burning-Mouth-Disease-Like Symptoms

3

3.1 Introduction

There are many reported causes of burning sensations of the mouth. However, these sensations are different from the ones described in Chap. 2. Therefore, such diseases and events cannot be considered true causes of BMD. Nevertheless, these diseases and events will be briefly mentioned in alphabetical order.

3.2 Allergy to Food Substances

In rare cases of BMD-like symptoms one may be dealing with allergy, for instance to peppermint oil, chewing gum, toothpaste, mouthrinses, lipstick and also cosmetic, and pharmaceutical products. Routine allergy testing in case of 'typical' BMD symptoms does not seem to be warranted.

3.3 Anaemia

Iron-deficiency is the most common cause of anaemia (see Glossary) and may cause BMD-like symptoms. Oral findings suggestive of the presence of iron-deficiency include cracks or fissures of the corners of the mouth and a smooth, red, painful

© The Author(s), under exclusive license to Springer Nature Switzerland AG 2022
I. van der Waal, *Burning Mouth Disease*,
https://doi.org/10.1007/978-3-030-94226-7_3

tongue. These signs and symptoms actually exclude a diagnosis of BMD.

Another cause of anaemia is a lack of vitamin B12. Oral symptoms may consist of a burning or itching sensation of the mucosa, taste disturbance, intolerance to wearing dentures, and, occasionally, dryness of the mouth. The tongue may obtain a smooth, fiery-red surface, being very different from the normal looking mucosa in BMD patients.

3.4   Blood Disorders

In a study among BMD patients no difference between the BMD group and the control group was found in routine blood analyses, including white blood cell count, red blood cell count, haemoglobin, and platelet count. Although several authors have reported opposite results, the relevance of routine blood analysis in BMD patients seems rather limited.

3.5   Dentures or Teeth Related Causes

3.5.1   Allergies to Dental Restorations

There have been some studies in patients suffering from BMD-like symptoms in whom hypersensitivity to dental restorations, e.g., amalgam fillings, has been demonstrated. However, the symptoms are very different from those of BMD.

3.5.2   Dental Treatment

Some BMD patients refer to recent dental treatment as the cause of their symptoms, as has been discussed in Chap. 2 under the heading of onset of symptoms. This belief applies to all types of dental treatment procedures, including root canal treatment and extraction of teeth. However, the scientific evidence is very weak and, therefore, dental treatment in BMD patients that is not truly indicated, is strongly discouraged. In some patients, such treatment may even worsen the symptoms.

3.5.3   Dentures

In the past, there was a strong belief that BMD was often caused by poor, ill-fitting dentures. Today that hypothesis is abandoned. In rare cases burning-mouth-disease-like symptoms are caused by an allergic reaction to acrylic substances in a denture.

3.6   Gastrointestinal Inflammation ('Gastritis')

Although gastrointestinal (see Glossary) inflammation occurs more often in BMD patients compared with healthy control subjects, it is unlikely that gastrointestinal problems are the cause of BMD and, therefore, routine referral of BMD patients, without symptoms of gastrointestinal disease, to a gastroenterologist does not seem to be warranted.

3.7   Hormonal Disorders

The rather strong preference of BMD for menopausal and postmenopausal women is suggestive of a gonodal (see Glossary) hormonal (estradiol and progesterone from the ovaries) disturbance in the development of BMD. However, hormonal replacement therapy has not shown to be of any benefit for women suffering from BMD.

3.8   Medication, Side Effects

Elderly people, being the largest group that is affected by BMD, often use several medications. The reduced physiologic reserve may make this group vulnerable to the noxious effects of medication. In view of the contradictory scientific results of various studies on this subject, there is insufficient support for the hypothesis that BMD is caused by any type of medication.

3.9   Mucosal Diseases

3.9.1   Cancer of the Mouth

Cancer of the mouth is very rare. The symptoms of such cancer vary widely, but localized burning or itching sensations may be the first symptoms. Typically, these sensations occur locally, one-sided, being very different from the two-sided burning sensations in BMD.

3.9.2   Candidiasis

Candidiasis is an inflammatory disease caused by a fungus, giving rise to whitish or reddish changes of the mucosa. Such changes of the oral mucosa are not compatible with a diagnosis of BMD. Also the symptoms associated with this fungal disease are very different from those of BMD.

3.9.3   Tongue Diseases

3.9.3.1   Coated or Hairy Tongue

A coated aspect of the surface of the tongue is rather common and is actually not based on a disease. In some cases, even hairlike, yellowish, or even black coating may occur (Fig. 3.1). Patients may or may not complain of some discomfort or a faulty taste. These symptoms are very different from those of BMD.

3.9.3.2   Fissured Tongue

Fissuring (formation of grooves) in the surface of the tongue is quite common and is not based on a disease. Few patients may experience some discomfort, being very different from the symptoms of BMD (Fig. 3.2).

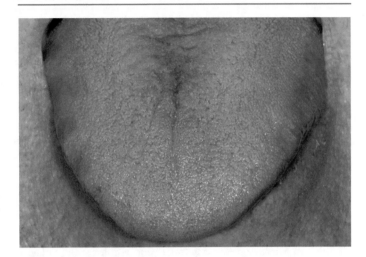

Fig. 3.1 Slightly coated tongue, not being the cause of BMD

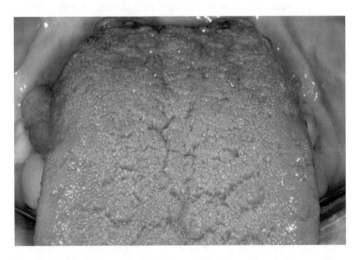

Fig. 3.2 Several grooves in the surface of the tongue ('fissured tongue'); are not the cause of BMD

3.9.3.3 Geographic Tongue

A map-like aspect ('geographic') of the mucosal surface of the tongue is called a geographic tongue (GT). It is a harmless, rather common condition of unknown aetiology (see Glossary), being characterized by recurrent smooth areas of the mucosa, surrounded by a whitish collar. Geographic tongue is often asymptomatic, and many patients are even not aware of the condition. Some patients, however, may experience burning sensations correlating well with the clinically visible changes of the lingual surface, but being quite different from BMD symptoms (Fig. 3.3).

3.10   Neurologic and Psychiatric Diseases

In the past, there was a strong belief that burning mouth disease (BMD) was caused by psychiatric diseases such as depression, anxiety, stress, and cancerophobia (exaggerated fear of suffering from cancer). The present view is, that BMD is most likely caused

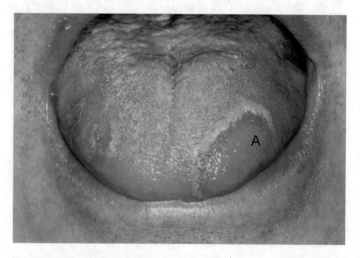

Fig. 3.3 In the anterior part of the coated tongue there is a smooth, red area (A), surrounded by a whitish collar, being diagnostic of geographic tongue; these changes are not the cause of BMD

by an altered function of the nerves. What causes this alteration and why it particularly affects the tongue is unknown. In fact, BMD may be regarded primarily as a chronic neuropathic pain.

The common association of BMD and signs of psychiatric diseases, such as depression and anxiety, can possibly be explained as being the result—and not the cause—of the miserable symptoms of BMD. Another possible explanation is a common pathway in the development of some psychiatric diseases and BMD.

3.11   Parafunctional Habits

Oral parafunctional habits refer to chronic, habitual chewing on the cheek or the lips. Another example of a parafunctional habit is tongue thrusting, where the tip of the tongue is continuously being pressed against the upper or lower teeth. Yet another parafunctional habit is bruxism ('grinding of the teeth'), particularly during sleep. There have been a few studies reported in which oral parafunctional habits were suggested to play a role in development of BMD. Yet, other authors have not been able to support this view.

3.12   Smoking and the Use of Alcohol

Smoking does not seem to play a role in the development of BMD. Nevertheless, some patients report that smoking aggravates the symptoms. The same experience applies to the use of alcohol.

3.13   Vitamin Deficiencies

The results of various studies on vitamin deficiencies in BMD patients have shown contradictory results. Nevertheless, some patients have been reported in whom suppletion of vitamin C improved the symptoms of BMD.

Reported Treatment Modalities of Burning Mouth Disease

4

4.1 Introduction

Since the aetiology of burning mouth disease (BMD) is unknown, treatment can only be symptomatic, being directed at alleviation of the symptoms. The reported treatments can be largely divided in (1) treatment with drugs, (2) alternative treatments, e.g., using herbal compounds, (3) treatment without drugs but with other means, e.g., acupuncture or soft laser, and (4) psychosocial intervention. In some cases the various treatment modalities can be combined, e.g., treatment with drugs supported by psychosocial interventions.

In the design of scientific studies on the efficacy of any type of treatment, one needs to include a *placebo* group, but only with consent of the patient. A placebo effect refers to the tendency of any medication, or other treatments, to exhibit positive results simply because the patient believes that it will work.(en.wikipedia.org) In a placebo structured study, the patients, and preferably also the doctors, should at the beginning of the study not be informed on which patients belong to the study group and which patients to the placebo group ('sham' group). This information should only be disclosed at the end of the study, allowing to objectively assess the efficacy of the treatment. In assessing the results of treatment, there may be also *nocebo* effects, being adverse effects from treatments that are

I. van der Waal, *Burning Mouth Disease*,
https://doi.org/10.1007/978-3-030-94226-7_4

induced by patients' negative expectations. Other important aspects of scientific studies on treatment results are the (small) number of patients included in the study and the (short) length of the study. For instance, some studies last only for a few months, while other studies have been performed during several years.

There is no internationally accepted standardization of how treatment results should be reported. As a result, it is often difficult, if not impossible, to compare the outcomes of the numerous studies on treatment of BMD.

4.2   Treatment with Drugs

4.2.1   Anaesthetic Lozenges; Paracetamol

In a short-term study of a small series of BMD patients, lozenges (sucking tablets) containing an anaesthetic (see Glossary) drug significantly reduced the burning oral pain and improved taste disturbances, but did not affect the feeling of a dry mouth. No long-term results have been reported.

Paracetamol, a well-known pain killer, is rarely effective in alleviating the burning symptoms in BMD patients, not even for a few hours.

4.2.2   Antidepressant, Antipsychotic, and Anxiolytic Drugs

4.2.2.1 Antidepressant Drugs

Antidepressant drugs are primarily used in the treatment of mood disorders. They have also been used in the treatment of neuropathic pain, including BMD. Although some positive results have been reported in the treatment of BMD, either alone or in combination with other measures, the use of antidepressants is somewhat limited because of adverse side effects such as dry mouth, drowsiness, and weight gain.

4.2.2.2 Antipsychotic Drugs

There are numerous antipsychotic drugs that have been used in the management of BMD patients, either alone or in combination with other measures. Unfortunately, there are no long-term studies reported.

4.2.2.3 Anxiolytic Drugs

Benzodiazepines, also referred to as 'Downers', have been mentioned as one of the few indications for management of chronic pain in general, not specifically focused on BMD. Clonazepam is one of the many subclasses of benzodiazepines that have been studied in the treatment of BMD. This drug can be applied topically in the mouth, e.g., sucking on one or more tablets per day, or by swallowing the drug ('systemic administration') during a number of weeks. When used systemically, side effects such as drowsiness and fatigue may occur, while in long-term use tolerance and dependence may occur. The results of the various studies on the use of anxiolytic drugs are somewhat controversial.

4.2.2.4 Comments

It is important to know that the prescription of antidepressant, antipsychotic, and anxiolytic drugs is not based on the hypothesis of BMD being primarily a psychiatric disease, but that such drugs may be helpful in tolerating the symptoms of BMD.

4.2.3 Capsaicin

Capsaicin is a molecule that is contained in hot peppers. It has been reported in short-term studies, either in the form of a mouthrinse or a topical gel, to have a favourable effect in the treatment of BMD. When used as an orally taken tablet, favourable results have been reported over a period of just 1 month. However, a substantial number of patients suffered from gastric pain.

4.2.4   Gonadal Hormones (Progesterone and Estrogens)

As has been mentioned already in Chap. 3, hormonal replacement therapy has not shown to be of much benefit for women suffering from BMD.

4.3   Alternative Treatments

4.3.1   Chewing Gum

Many BMD patients favour the use of chewing gum to alleviate their symptoms. There is scientific support for the use of chewing gum in BMD patients, particularly when associated with xerostomia. Some patients reject the use of chewing because of a 'bad appearance'.

4.3.2   Herbal Compounds

There are many herbal compounds that have been used for the treatment of chronic pain, including BMD. Just a few examples of such compounds will be discussed.

4.3.2.1 Aloe Vera

Aloe vera grows wild in tropical climates around the world and is cultivated for agricultural and medicinal uses. There is hardly any clinical evidence for the effectiveness or safety for its use as a medicine. This also applies to its use in BMD.

4.3.2.2 Alpha-Lipoic Acid

Alpha-lipoic acid (ALA) is a vitamin-like substance that can be found in foods, such as spinach, broccoli, potatoes, and organ meats, such as liver. In some countries ALA is available as an over-the-counter nutritional supplement as a tablet or a capsule. There is limited evidence of a positive effect of ALA on any disease, including BMD.

4.3.2.3 Chamomile
One of the most common herbs used for medicinal purposes is chamomile, whose standardized tea and herbal extracts are prepared from dried flowers of *Matricaria* species. Chamomile has pain-killing and anti-inflammatory properties. However, the general view is that there is no scientific evidence that chamomile has any effect beneficial on health or diseases.

4.3.2.4 Kampo Medicines
In a study from Japan, favourable results of the treatment of BMD have been reported by the use of Kampo medicines (Sai-boku-to). To the best of my knowledge, no studies on this herbal compound have been reported outside Japan.

4.3.3   Homeopathy

There is just one BMD patient reported who has been successfully treated with homeopathy.

4.4   Treatment Without Drugs

4.4.1   Acupuncture

There are a few reports, particularly from China, of positive results of the use of acupuncture in the management of BMD patients. However, the scientific evidence of the validity of this type of treatment is weak.

4.4.2   Blockade of Nerves; Surgical Interruption of Neural Structures

There is not much evidence that blockade of certain nerves by injection of anaesthetic solutions is useful in the management of BMD. The same holds true for attempts to surgically interrupt the neural structures. In fact, such irreversible procedures may worsen the symptoms. Therefore, such treatments should be discouraged.

4.4.3   Electromagnetic Millimetre Wave Therapy

Electromagnetic millimetre wave therapy (EMVT) is a noninvasive technique, consisting of the exposure of parts of the human body to electromagnetic radiation. Based on a study among 80 BMD patients in China, the authors hypothesized that EMVT may become a new treatment method for BMD patients. In the Western world EMVT has not gained much acceptance, mainly because of the lack of an accepted mechanism explaining how EMVT can be therapeutic.

4.4.4   Low-Level Laser Therapy

Low-level laser therapy (LLLT), also referred to as 'soft laser', is a form of medicine that applies low-level (low-power) lasers. The reported results of LLLT in the management of BMD are rather contradictory.

4.4.5   Tongue Protector

In some studies positive results have been reported by the use of a tongue protector (a transparent polyethylene sheath covering the tongue from the tip to the posterior part), in order to avoid continuous rubbing of the tongue against the teeth or the dentures. However, the scientific evidence of its use is weak.

4.5   Psychosocial Intervention; Cognitive Behavioural Therapy

It is well known that BMD may be associated with psychogenic disorders, such as anxiety and depression. However, patients' acceptance of a possibly associated psychogenic disorder can be a major hurdle. Furthermore, there are no convincing studies that support the value of psychosocial intervention in BMD patients.

Patients who have become depressed or anxious due to the symptoms of BMD might be referred to a cognitive behavioural therapist. Cognitive behavioural therapy is directed at influencing patterns of thinking or behaviour in order to accept and cope with the problems that patients are faced with. Unfortunately, good-quality studies are lacking.

4.6   Summarizing Conclusion

Based on several reviews of the literature, the conclusion can be drawn that there is insufficient scientific evidence to support or refute the use of any interventions in managing BMD [20]. In other words, there is no proven treatment that will be effective in each BMD patient. In spite of the lack of scientific evidence, some treatments may be effective in one patient, while they are not in another patient. Furthermore, favourable results have been reported on a combination of various treatments, e.g., the use of a tongue protector and Aloe vera. Anyhow, one should avoid irreversible treatments, such as cutting of nerves or extraction of one or more teeth.

Ideally, patients and doctors should discuss with each other which treatment or combination of treatments may be worth trying ('shared decision').

Management of Burning Mouth Disease

5

5.1 Introduction

The low prevalence of burning mouth disease (BMD) and the complexity of the symptoms require a multidisciplinary approach (doctors and dentists with various backgrounds) to properly diagnose and manage the patients suffering from this disease. It is a challenge to bring healthcare providers together who have the expertise to participate in such a multidisciplinary team, either working together in a single healthcare institution or spread over different dental or medical offices. Although the final outcome of a multidisciplinary approach may still be limited, it avoids the patients from being transferred from one doctor to the other. Furthermore, there is the advantage for the patient of being managed by dentists and doctors who are well acquainted with BMD.

For less experienced first-line healthcare workers the symptoms of BMD may not be recognized immediately. As a result, various diagnostic tests and treatments may be carried out that are not truly indicated. This also applies to random, unfocused referrals to other doctors.

© The Author(s), under exclusive license to Springer Nature
Switzerland AG 2022
I. van der Waal, *Burning Mouth Disease*,
https://doi.org/10.1007/978-3-030-94226-7_5

5.2   Oral Examination

There are many oral lesions and conditions that may produce BMD-like symptoms, as has been discussed in Chap. 3. Since most general practitioners have hardly been trained in performing an oral examination, such examination should preferably be in the hands of a healthcare provider with a dental background.

For the patient it is often difficult to understand when, on professional inspection of the tongue or other burning parts of the mouth, no abnormalities can be seen ("Do you really not see anything abnormal on my tongue"? or "My tongue looks very strange"), particularly in the presence of harmless, not BMD-related coating or fissuring of the tongue (see Chap. 3).

5.3   Laboratory Investigations

5.3.1 Laboratory Investigations

In the absence of oral lesions, a number of items need to be taken into account:

1. Cytological (see Glossary) or histological (see Glossary) examination of clinically normal mucosa may have some scientific value but rarely contributes to the management of a patient suffering from BMD. The same applies to taking cultures (smears) for the demonstration of fungi or other microorganisms, e.g., *Candida albicans*.
2. Investigation for allergy for dental materials is rarely helpful; the same applies for allergy for food substances.
3. Measuring the salivary secretion and the composition of saliva rarely contributes to the management of BMD. The same applies for testing smell or taste.
4. The results of blood examination, of whatever type, including examination for vitamin deficiencies, will rarely, if ever, contribute to the management of a BMD patient.

5. Although a few authors recommend including investigation of thyroid function in the diagnostic process of all BMD patients, the general view is that such evaluation is not relevant for the management of BMD.
6. Neurological examination, including CT or MRI-imaging of the brain, is rarely, if ever, of relevance for the management of the patient.

5.4   Dental Treatment

Since BMD is not caused by dental faults, one should avoid dental treatment, e.g., replacement of dental restorations or even extraction of one or more teeth. In fact, such dental treatments may even worsen the symptoms ("Doctor, when I came to your office I had a severe problem, but I could manage it. Now you have treated me, my problem has become worse; what have you done?").

5.5   The Importance of Proper Communication

In a study in the U.K., the experience and understanding of chronic pain in and around the mouth, including a number of BMD patients, was evaluated among patients and medical and dental healthcare providers [21]. One of the observations was that patients often get the impression of being passed between dental and medical services (sent 'from pillar to post') that have limited interaction. They may feel unsupported by both dental and medical health services. Another interesting finding of this study was, that both dentists and GPs experienced interactions with patients as frustrating and demanding to manage, seeing this effort as undervalued and time-consuming.

The importance of proper communication between healthcare professionals and patients has been well documented in a study among chronic pain patients and their pain specialist [22]. In this study, an implicit dialogue between doctors (often adhering to a psychogenic model) and their patients (usually adhering to a somatic (see Glossary) model) was identified that appeared to undermine the quality of their interactions, challenged each other's credibility and caused distress to both parties.

In view of the complexity of BMD the spouse or a close relative or friend should be present during the dialogue with the healthcare provider.

5.6   Patient Information

Proper information about BMD is usually a big relief for the patients, because (1) BMD is an accepted disease; it has a name, and the patient is apparently not the only one suffering from this disease, (2) dentists and doctors that have been consulted in the past may have told the patient, erroneously so, that the symptoms are caused by an underlying psychiatric illness. To hear that such information is not correct, is usually very important for the patients, since they often have felt to be regarded by their doctors as a 'psychiatric' case, and (3) the disease is not life-threatening and is not a sign of an underlying cancer, sometimes resulting in the patient saying: "What a relief, I was really afraid of having cancer. Now I know that it is a harmless disease, I think I can live with it."

It should be made clear that, in view of the poorly understood aetiology of BMD, treatment can, at best, only be symptomatic and may somewhat alleviate the symptoms, not curing the disease Just bluntly telling the patients that 'nothing can be done' is for most patients a great deception [23].

A patient may need a time-out, e.g., of a few weeks, to 'digest' all the information before taking a decision on further steps in the management. Preferably, any decision on management should be a 'shared decision' between doctor and patient.

After being informed about the various aspects of BMD, many patients do not insist on any further treatment. A number of these patients happily accept a proposal for regular follow-up visits, e.g., at six or 12 month intervals, while others question the value of such follow-up visits ("What is the use of coming back in the absence of effective treatment"?).

In spite of being informed about the lack of effective diagnostic tests and therapeutic measures, some patients will insist on treatment and further diagnostic tests. From a doctors' point of view it seems acceptable to give in to the patient's request to some extent, e.g., for doing blood examination.

A few patients will be disappointed and sometimes even angry ("I thought that you were going to take care of my problem, but apparently you cannot; did I have to travel all this way just to hear this"?), being not interested in any further communication.

Some BMD patients have fixed beliefs about their disease based on information from websites, not realizing that such information may be of questionable quality [24].

5.7   Various Treatment Modalities

An overview of the various treatment modalities, as being discussed in Chap. 4, has been presented in Table 5.1. Based on several critical reviews of the literature, the conclusion can be drawn that there is insufficient scientific evidence to support or refute the use of any medication and other interventions in managing BMD. In other words, there is no treatment that will be effective in each BMD patient. Nevertheless, certain treatments or combinations of treatments may be effective in some patients, while they are not in others. At any rate, one should avoid irreversible treatments, such as cutting of nerves or extraction of one or more teeth.

In view of the numerous treatment modalities discussed in Chap. 4, it is obvious that no single specialist, nor any pain clinic, will have the facilities and the expertise to offer all these modalities to BMD patients. For instance, some clinicians or pain clinics may favour low-level laser therapy, while others will never use this modality. As has been mentioned already in the previous chapter, patients and doctors should discuss with each other which treatment or combination of treatments may be worth trying ('shared decision').

Table 5.1 Treatment modalities in burning mouth disease

Treatment with drugs
1. Anaesthetic lozenges and paracetamol
2. Antidepressant drugs
3. Antipsychotic drugs
4. Anxiolytic drugs
5. Capsaicin
6. Gonadal hormones (progesterone, estrogens and testosterone)

Alternative treatments
1. Chewing gum
2. Herbal compounds
3. Homeopathy

Treatment without drugs
1. Acupuncture
2. Blockade of nerves
3. Electromagnetic millimetre wave therapy
4. Low-level laser therapy
5. Tongue protector

Psychosocial intervention; cognitive behavioural therapy

General practitioners seem to be 'well prepared' to prescribe drugs for the management of chronic neuropathic pain in general. On the other hand, dentists are less well prepared to prescribe this type of medication. In such event, the dentist may ask the general practitioner to take care of the medication. In this way, the number of unnecessary referrals to secondary healthcare providers may be reduced.

5.8   Self-Care

Many patients have found some way already to alleviate their symptoms, e.g., by the avoidance of spicy food. Some patients benefit from sugar-free chewing gum, while others reject the use of chewing gum, mainly because of a 'bad appearance'. The daily use of oral lubricants or chamomile mouthrinses (see Chap. 4) may be helpful in some patients, while others feel relieved by rinsing their mouth with over-the-counter saliva formulations or the use of sialogogues, e.g., lemon drops, to increase the production of saliva. Yet others prefer the use of carbonated soft drinks or sucking on ice cubes.

In case of abnormal or complete absence of taste, BMD patients may benefit from over-the-counter available nutritional supplements, such as alpha-lipoic acid. There are no effective means to improve any smell disorders that may be associated with BMD.

5.9   Psychosocial Intervention; Cognitive Behavioural Therapy

As discussed in Chap. 4, there is insufficient evidence to support or refute the use of any interventions in managing BMD, including psychosocial intervention and cognitive behavioural therapy. Actually as with all types of treatments, that have been discussed, some patients want to try it and may benefit from such interventions. Others just refuse such intervention, simply because they have fixed beliefs in a somatic cause of BMD, sometimes saying "I am not crazy".

5.10   Referral to a Specialist or a Multidisciplinary Pain Clinic

When a primary healthcare worker or the patient feels the need for referral to a specialist or a multidisciplinary pain clinic, the clinician should help the patient to avoid of getting lost in a doctor's circuit ('doctor shopping'), being transferred from one to the other. The patient should be offered the opportunity to stay in touch with the referring dentists or general practitioner, thereby preventing the patients' feeling of getting lost in a merry-go-round. Patients should only be referred to a specialist who has experience with managing patients suffering from BMD, thereby avoiding a disappointment for the patient. Furthermore, the patient's expectations of a consultation should not be raised too high, avoiding saying: "I know a specialist who is very knowledgeable and who will take care of your problem". This may only aggravate the disappointment when no solution of the problem can be offered.

5.11   A Letter from a Patient

The following letter, that I received by e-mail from a BMD patient, well describes the complaints that patients can be faced with and their way of trying to cope with the disease: "I am a 57-year-old woman and since 1 year I have been suffering from unbearable complaints in my mouth. It is difficult to describe these complaints. Words like 'pressing pain', 'current', 'burning', 'radiating pain' from my tongue and my palate to the upper teeth and, sometimes, also to the face around my nose somewhat cover these complaints. They vary in intensity and increase in the course of the day and become worse while speaking, eating, and drinking.

There are no problems in my personal life. I am married with three beautiful daughters. In the past year, I have visited my general practitioner, my dentist, an oral and maxillofacial surgeon, a physiotherapist specialized in chronic head-and-neck pain disorders, a gastroenterologist and an ENT doctor. Blood examination and endoscopies have not revealed any abnormalities. Finally, a diagnosis of 'neuropathic symptoms, compatible with burning mouth disease' has been rendered. In the absence of measures to cure this disease, I have accepted the suggestion to try to cope with my symptoms and I have been supported by a psychologist. Unfortunately, the quality of my life remains poor. If you have no suggestions for any further examinations or treatment, just let me know. I am not insisting on any redundant investigations or treatments. Furthermore, I truly trust the various healthcare providers that I have been visiting. However, I just want to be sure that I collected as much information as possible about this disease". This letter well describes the despair of the patient. At the same time, her rational approach is remarkable and may not be expected from each BMD patient.

5.12 Patient Support Groups

In several countries in the world, a society have been set up to support BMD patients. There is also a Facebook group on this subject (https://www.facebook.com/groups/burningmouth-syndrome).

5.13 Future Perspectives

Financial support for studies on BMD is limited due to the rarity of the disease. Besides, BMD is not a life-threatening disease. Nevertheless, several studies in different parts of the world are in progress, focusing on a better understanding of the disease and the development of new treatment modalities.

5.14 Postscriptum

It is well recognized that the author's experience is limited to patients living in a country in the Western World. Management of patients suffering from BMD may, indeed, be different in various parts of the world, e.g., relating to patients' expectations from dental and medical care and the accessibility of such care. In addition, there may be differences between patients' expectations and needs between those who live in rural areas and those who live in large communities.

It is the author's experience that proper patient information and empathy will often change an apparently unbearable disease into a more or less acceptable one to live with, thereby avoiding redundant dental or medical treatments, drug prescriptions, and referrals.

Glossary

Aetiology   the cause of a disease

Anaemia   is a condition in which there are not sufficient healthy red blood cells to carry adequate oxygen to your body's tissues

Buccal (mucosa)   the inner side of the cheek

Cytological   related to the various aspects of cells in the human body

Comorbidity   the presence of two or more diseases in the same person

Dysaesthesia   an abnormal sensation

Epidemiology   describes the various demographic aspects of a disease, such as the prevalence (how frequent does the disease occur among the population), age and gender of affected people, possible geographic differences, and the way of spreading of an infectious disease in various parts of the world

Extraoral   outside the mouth

Gastrointestinal   relating to the stomach (gastric) and the intestines (bowel)

Gonodal hormones   female sex hormones are produced in the ovaries

Histological   related to the various aspects of tissues in the human body

Intraoral   in the mouth

Mucosa   the moist, inner lining (comparable to the skin) of body cavities, such as the mouth (oral mucosa)

© The Editor(s) (if applicable) and The Author(s), under exclusive license to Springer Nature Switzerland AG 2022
I. van der Waal, *Burning Mouth Disease*,
https://doi.org/10.1007/978-3-030-94226-7

Prevalence   the proportion of persons in a population who have a particular disease at a specified point in time (e.g. today). For instance, the number of people that suffer today from burning mouth disease

Somatic disease   a disease of the body

Temporomandibular joint disorder   a malfunction of the joint between the temporal bone of the skull and the mandibular bone (= lower jaw)

References

1. Périer JM, Boucher Y. History of burning mouth syndrome (1800-1950): a review. Oral Dis. 2019;25(2):425–38. https://doi.org/10.1111/odi.12860.
2. Lamey PJ, Lamb AB, Hughes A, Milligan KA, Forsyth A. Type 3 burning mouth syndrome: psychological and allergic aspects. J Oral Pathol Med. 1994;23:216–9.
3. Scala A, Checchi L, Montevecchi M, Marini I, Giamberardino MA. Update on burning mouth syndrome: overview and patient management. Crit Rev Oral Biol Med. 2003;14(4):275–91.
4. Kohorst JJ, Bruce AJ, Torgerson RR, Schenck LA, Davis MD. A population-based study of the incidence of burning mouth syndrome. Mayo Clin Proc. 2014;89(11):1545–52. https://doi.org/10.1016/j.mayocp.2014.05.018.
5. Bergdahl M, Bergdahl J. Burning mouth syndrome: prevalence and associated factors. J Oral Pathol Med. 1999 Sep;28(8):350–4.
6. Tarkkila L, Linna M, Tiitinen A, Lindqvist C, Meurman JH. Oral symptoms at menopause--the role of hormone replacement therapy. Oral Surg Oral Med Oral Pathol Oral Radiol Endod. 2001;92(3):276–80.
7. Moore PA, Guggenheimer J, Orchard T. Burning mouth syndrome and peripheral neuropathy in patients with type 1 diabetes mellitus. J Diabetes Complicat. 2007;21(6):397–402.
8. Wang H, He F, Xu C, Fang C, Peng J. Clinical analysis for oral mucosal disease in 21 972 cases. Zhong Nan Da Xue Xue Bao Yi Xue Ban. 2018;43(7):779–83. https://doi.org/10.11817/j.issn.1672-7347.2018.07.013. (Article in Chinese).
9. Wolf E, Birgerstam P, Nilner M, Petersson K. Nonspecific chronic orofacial pain: studying patient experiences and perspectives with a qualitative approach. J Orofac Pain. 2008;22(4):349–58.
10. Oghli I, List T, Su N, Häggman-Henrikson B. The impact of orofacial pain conditions on oral health related quality of life: a systematic review. J Oral Rehabil. 2020;47(8):1052–64. https://doi.org/10.1111/joor.12994.

© The Editor(s) (if applicable) and The Author(s), under exclusive
license to Springer Nature Switzerland AG 2022
I. van der Waal, *Burning Mouth Disease*,
https://doi.org/10.1007/978-3-030-94226-7

11. Pereira JV, Normando AGC, Rodrigues-Fernandes CI, Rivera C, Santos-Silva AR, Lopes MA. The impact on quality of life in patients with burning mouth syndrome: a systematic review and meta-analysis. Oral Surg Oral Med Oral Pathol Oral Radiol. 2021;131(2):186–94. https://doi.org/10.1016/j.oooo.2020.11.019.

12. van der Ploeg HM, van der Wal N, Eijkman MAJ, van der Waal I. Psychological aspects of patients with burning mouth syndrome. Oral Surg Oral Med Oral Pathol. 1987;63(6):664–8.

13. Grushka M. Clinical features of burning mouth syndrome. Oral Surg Oral Med Oral Pathol. 1987;63(1):30–6.

14. López-Jornet P, Molino-Pagan D, Andujar Mateos P, Rodriguez Agudo C, Pons-Fuster A. Circadian rhythms variation of pain in burning mouth syndrome. Geriatr Gerontol Int. 2015;15(4):490–5. https://doi.org/10.1111/ggi.12303.

15. Sardella A, Lodi G, Demarosi F, Bez C, Cassano S, et al. Burning mouth syndrome: a retrospective study investigating spontaneous remission and response to treatments. Oral Dis. 2006;12(2):152–5.

16. Hampf G. Dilemma in treatment of patients suffering from orofacial dysaesthesia. Int J Oral Maxillofac Surg. 1987;16(4):397–401.

17. Corsalini M, Di Venere D, Pettini F, Lauritano D, Petruzzi M. Temporomandibular disorders in burning mouth syndrome patients: an observational study. Int J Med Sci. 2013;10(12):1784–9. https://doi.org/10.7150/ijms.6327.

18. Mignogna MD, Pollio A, Fortuna G, Leuci S, Ruoppo E, Adamo D, et al. Unexplained somatic comorbidities in patients with burning mouth syndrome: a controlled clinical study. J Orofac Pain. 2011;25(2):131–40.

19. Freilich JE, Kuten-Shorrer M, Treister NS, Woo SB, Villa A. Burning mouth syndrome: a diagnostic challenge. Oral Surg Oral Med Oral Pathol Oral Radiol. 2020;129(2):120–4. https://doi.org/10.1016/j.oooo.2019.09.015.

20. McMillan R, Forssell H, Buchanan JA, Glenny AM, Weldon JC, Zakrzewska JM. Interventions for treating burning mouth syndrome. Cochrane Database Syst Rev. 2016;11:CD002779.

21. Peters S, Goldthorpe J, McElroy C, King E, Javidi H, Tickle M, et al. Managing chronic orofacial pain: a qualitative study of patients', doctors', and dentists' experiences. Br J Health Psychol. 2015 Nov;20(4):777–91. https://doi.org/10.1111/bjhp.12141.

22. Kenny DT. Constructions of chronic pain in doctor-patient relationships: bridging the communication chasm. Patient Educ Couns. 2004;52(3):297–305.

23. Petrie KJ, Frampton T, Large RG, Moss-Morris R, Johnson M, Meechan G. What do patients expect from their first visit to a pain clinic? Clin J Pain. 2005;21(4):297–301.

24. Fortuna G, Schiavo JH, Aria M, Mignona MD, Klasser GD. The usefulness of You TubeTM as a source of information on burning mouth syndrome. J Oral Rehabil. 2019;46:657–65.

Printed in the United States
by Baker & Taylor Publisher Services